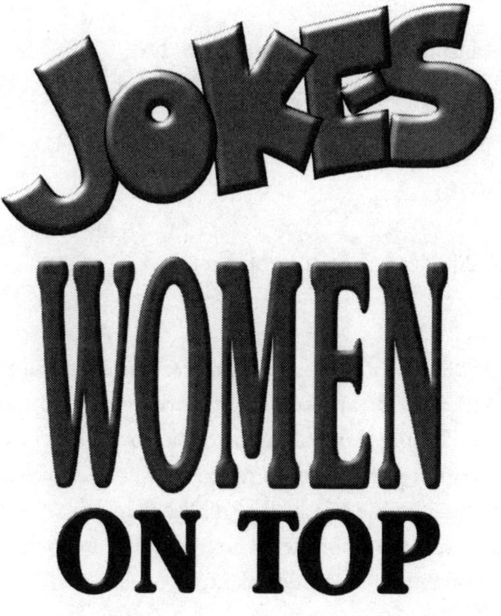

ON TOP

SUE PERIER

Strathearn Publishing

Strathearn Publishing
PO Box 44, Slough, Berkshire, SL1 4YN

Trade Distribution by W. Foulsham & Co. Ltd,
The Publishing House, Bennetts Close, Cippenham, Slough, Berkshire,
SL1 5AP, England

ISBN 0-572-02817-2

Printed in Great Britain by Cox & Wyman Ltd, Reading, Berkshire

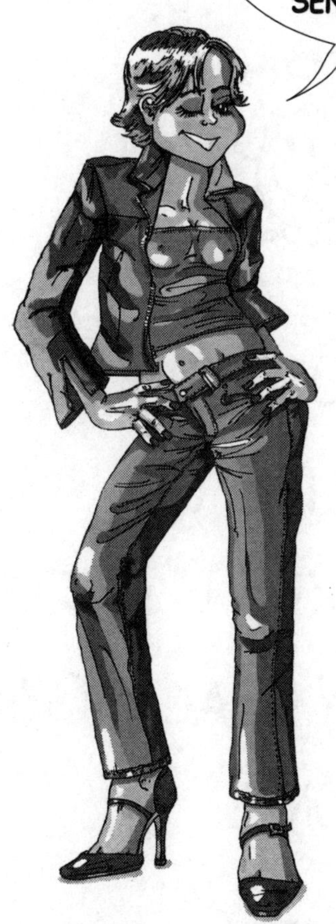
REMEMBER – NO-ONE EVER GOT LAID WEARING SENSIBLE SHOES!

WHY IS E-MAIL
LIKE A MAN'S DICK?

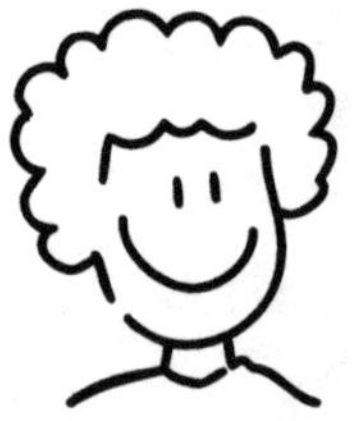

IT'S MORE FUN
WHEN IT'S UP,
BUT IT MAKES IT HARD
TO GET ANY REAL WORK
DONE.

WHY ARE MEN LIKE FRESHLY GROUND COFFEE?

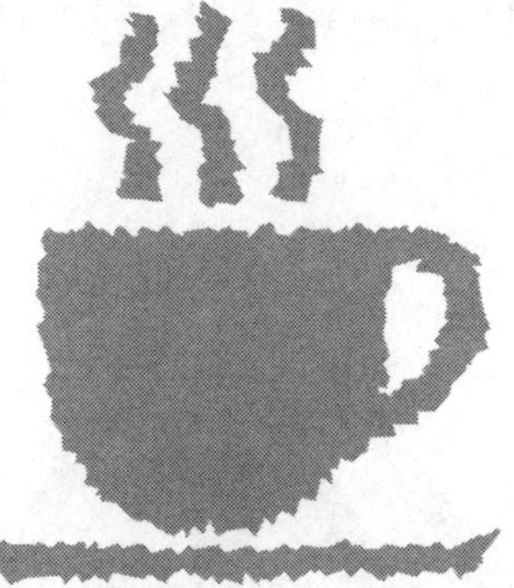

THE BEST ONES ARE RICH, WARM AND CAN KEEP YOU UP ALL NIGHT LONG.

Why does it take a million sperm to fertilise one egg?

They won't stop for directions.

What do you call a woman without an asshole?

Single.

Why does a man's penis have a hole in it?

So he can get oxygen to his brain.

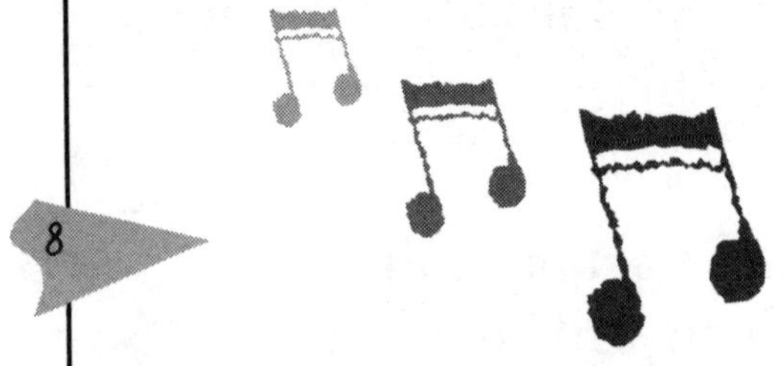

Why do men whistle
when they're sitting on the toilet?

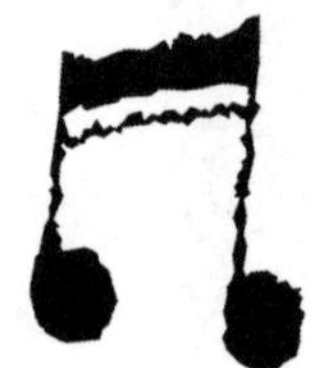

Because it helps them remember which end they need to wipe.

Ten things not to say when having sex

1 You woke me up for that?

2 I hope you're as good looking when I'm sober.

3 You're almost as good as my ex!

4 So much for the fulfilment of sexual fantasies!

5 Keep the noise down, my mother's a light sleeper.

6 But I just steam-cleaned this sofa!

7 I want a baby!

8 There's cobwebs on the lampshade.

9 Did I remember to take my pill?

END Now I know why she dumped you.

What did God say after he created man?

'I can do better than this!'

What is the difference between a Porsche and a hedgehog?

The hedgehog has pricks on the outside.

What goes in hard and pink, but comes out soft and mushy?

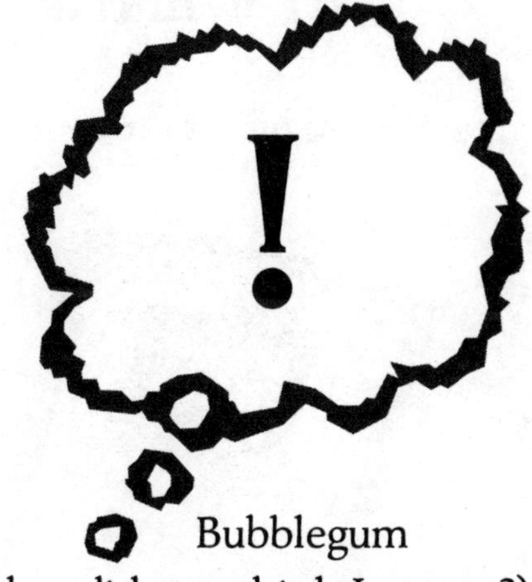

Bubblegum
(what did you think I meant?)

What is the difference between men and women?

A woman wants one man to satisfy her every need, while a man wants every woman to satisfy his one need.

How do you stop your husband reading your e-mails?

Rename the folder 'instruction manuals'.

If a guy tells you he's a perfect blend of the strong macho man with a sensitive feminine side – he's a gay lorry driver.

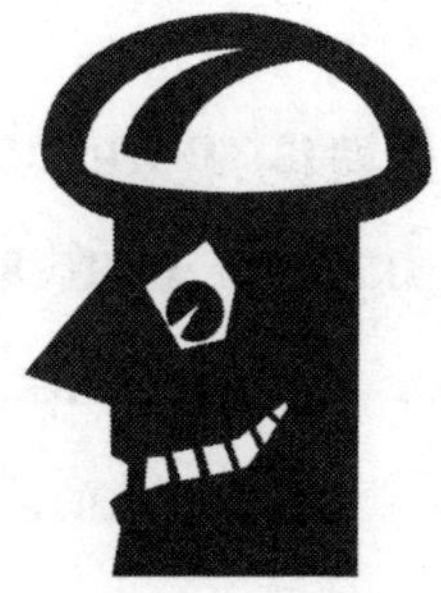

Why are men like bicycle helmets?

They are handy in an emergency, but otherwise they just look silly.

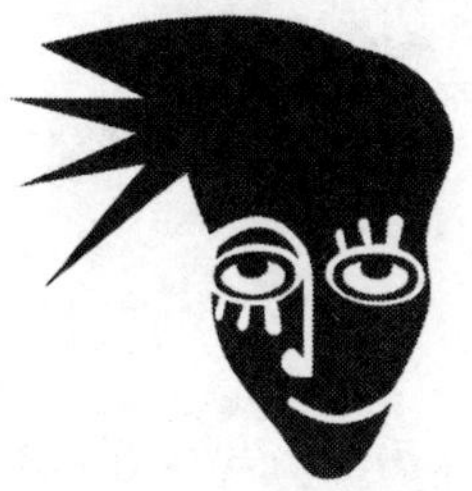

Why are men like mascara?

They run at the first sign of emotion.

Three old ladies were sitting on a park bench and a man jumped out of the bushes and flashed them.

Two of them had a stroke but the third one wasn't quick enough.

Any woman who thinks the way to a man's heart is through his stomach is aiming a little too high.

The trouble with some women is that they get all excited about nothing ...
and then they marry him.

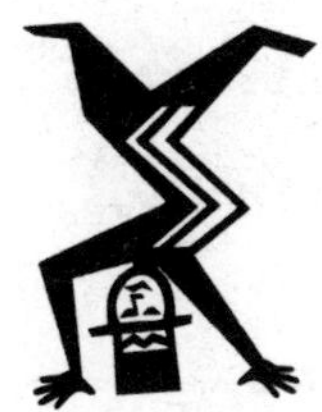

What's the definition of misogynist?
A man who hates every bone in a woman's body ...
except his own.

WHAT DO YOU DO WITH A MAN WHO THINKS HE'S GOD'S GIFT?

EXCHANGE HIM.

When a woman says:
'Come on! This place is a mess! You and I need to clean up. Your pants are on the floor and you'll have no clothes if we don't do the washing now!'

A man hears:
'Come on! ... blah, blah, blah ... you and I ... blah, blah, blah, blah, blah ... on the floor ... blah, blah, blah ... no clothes ... blah, blah, blah ... now!'

Why are men like new-born babies?

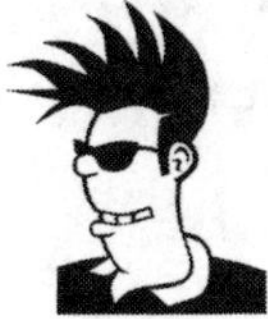
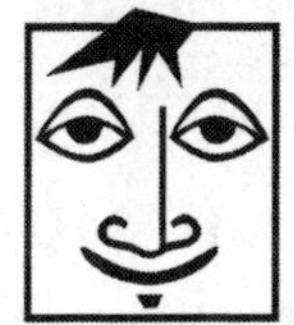
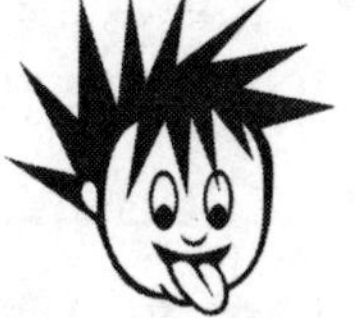

They're cute at first, but you soon get tired of cleaning up their crap.

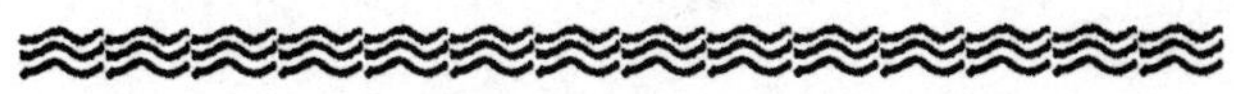

WHY ARE MEN LIKE LAXATIVES?

THEY IRRITATE THE SHIT OUT OF YOU.

A 54-year-old maths professor was having an affair with his 18-year-old teaching assistant. He thought his wife would be furious when she found out but she just smiled.

'I'm having an affair with an 18-year-old lifeguard,' she told him, 'and 18 goes into 54 more times than 54 goes into 18.'

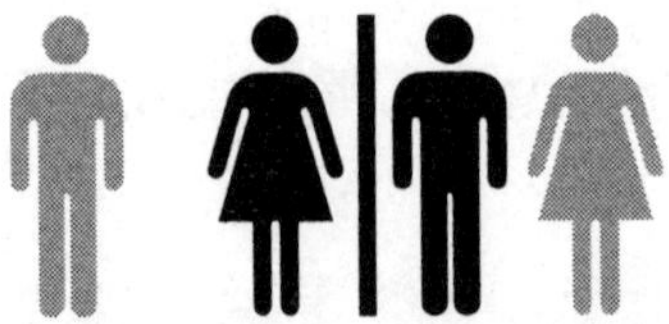

How many men does it take to put the toilet seat down?

Nobody knows, it hasn't happened yet.

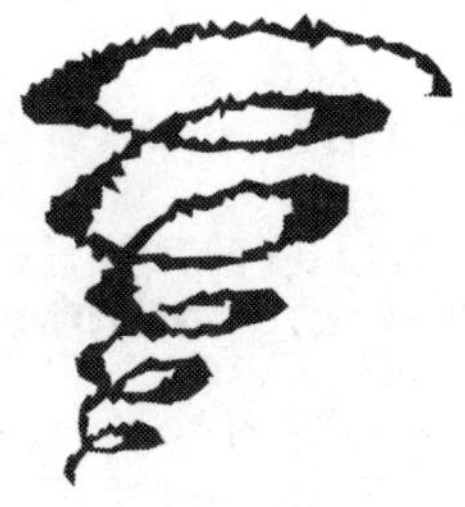

Why are men like blenders?

You think you need one, but you're not quite sure why.

Ten things not to say to a naked man:

1 This explains your car.

2 Ahh, it's cute.

3 I've smoked fatter joints than that.

4 Wow, and your feet are so big.

5 It's okay, we'll work around it.

6 Can I be honest with you?

7 How sweet, you brought incense.

8 Why don't we skip to the cigarettes?

9 It's a good thing you have so many other talents.

10 So this is why you're supposed to judge people on personality.

MASTURBATE

Why do men masturbate?

They like having sex with someone they love.

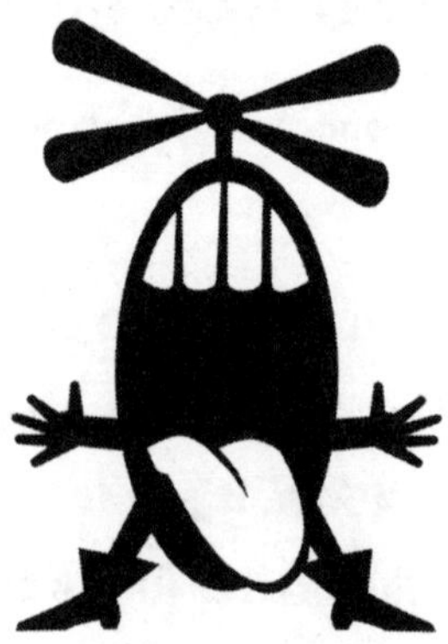

Why are men like Belgian chocolate?

They are sweet, smooth and they head straight for your hips.

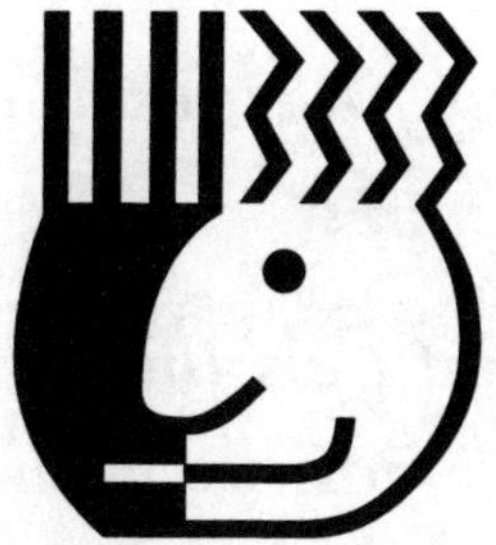

WHY IS IT SO HARD FOR WOMEN TO FIND SENSITIVE, CARING AND HANDSOME MEN?

THEY ALREADY HAVE BOYFRIENDS.

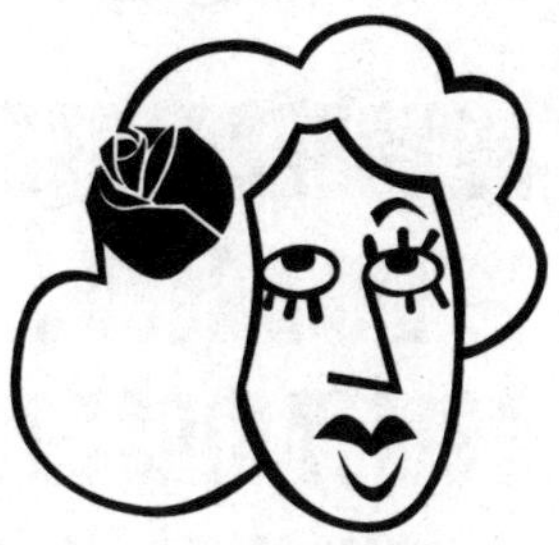

Why do most women fake orgasm?

Because most men fake foreplay.

How do you find out if a guy is intelligent?

Ask him what he's thinking about. If he's intelligent, he'll take a moment to reply because it's bound to be sex or football and he has to make up something else.

OF COURSE I DON'T
LOOK BUSY ...
I DID IT RIGHT THE
FIRST TIME.

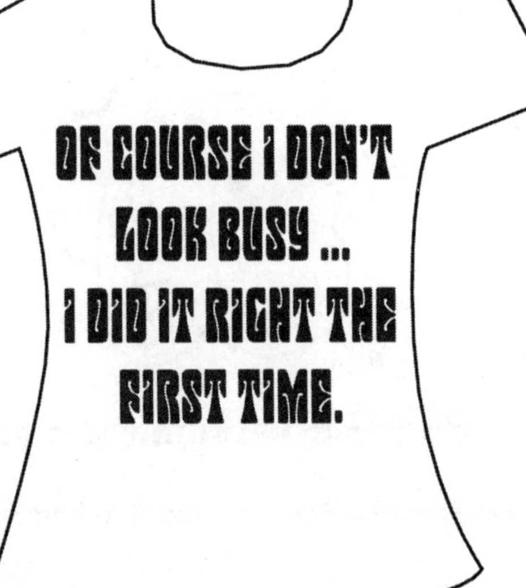

Why are men like carpets?

If you lay them right the first time, you can walk all over them for years!

Why did the man put 10p in his condom?

Because if he couldn't come, at least he could call.

Why are men like cut glass?

They look great but you can still see right through them.

Why was the guy disappointed when he bought a copy of *Women Who Love Too Much*?

It didn't have any phone numbers.

Why do midwives slap babies' bottoms as soon as they are born?

To knock the penises off the smart ones.

Why are men like high-heeled sandals?

They're easy to walk on once you get the hang of it.

Why is e-mail like a man's dick?
Because those who don't have it agree that it's useful, but think it's not worth the fuss that those who have it make about it.

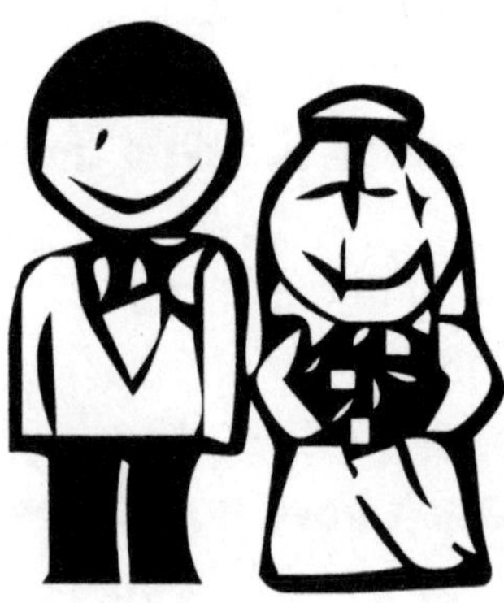

Where is the best place to find a man who is handsome, a good lover and a stimulating partner?

In a romantic novel.

A WOMAN'S GUIDE TO MEN'S ENGLISH

I'm hungry. = ***I'm hungry.***

I'm angry. = ***I'm angry.***

I'm tired. = ***I'm tired.***

Yes, I like the way you had your hair cut.
= ***You've had your hair cut?***

Nice dress! = ***Nice cleavage!***

I don't think that blouse and that skirt go well together.
= ***I'm gay.***

I like that one better.
= ***Pick any bloody dress and let's go!***

I'm going out with my mates.
= ***I'm going to get completely plastered.***

Do you want to watch a video?
= ***I fancy a night in and sex with you later.***

Do you want to go to the cinema?
= ***I fancy a night out and sex with you later.***

I'm bored. = ***Do you want to have sex?***

I love you. = ***Let's have sex now.***

What's wrong? = ***I don't see the problem – but I suppose sex tonight is out of the question?***

Let's talk. = ***If you think I'm a deep person, will you have sex with me?***

Will you marry me?= ***I don't want you to have sex with anyone else.***

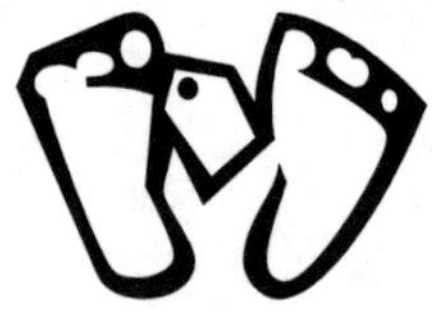

Why did God create man?

Because a vibrator can't put up shelves.

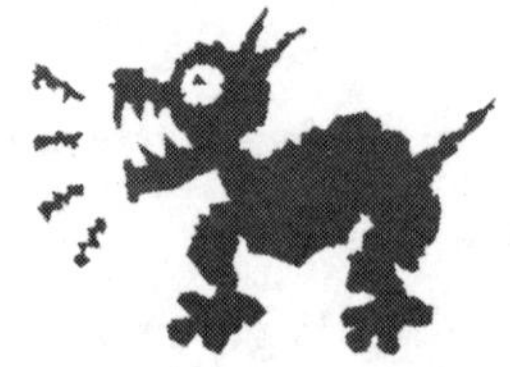

Why did God give men larger brains than dogs?

So they wouldn't hump women's legs at parties.

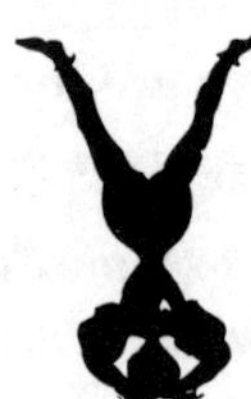

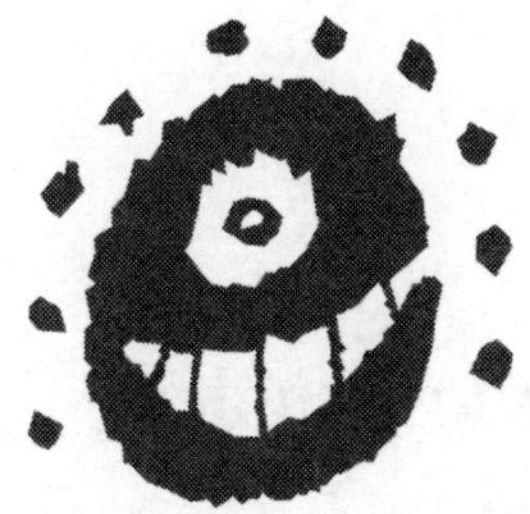

A Friend of mine got her Valium mixed up with her birth control pills.

She had 10 kids, but she couldn't give a damn.

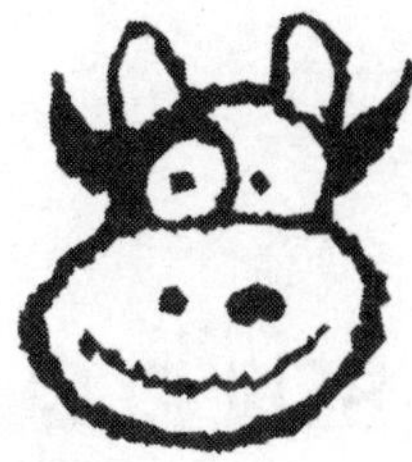

Sometimes I think I understand men, then I regain consciousness.

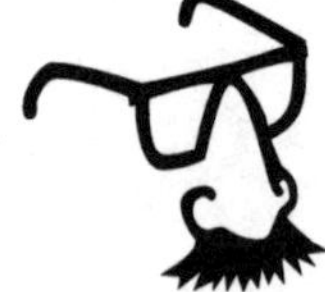

Why do female black widow spiders kill their males after mating?

To stop the snoring before it starts.

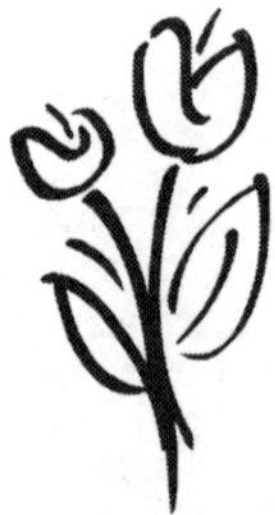

BEHIND EVERY SUCCESSFUL MAN IS A WOMAN SHOVELLING THE SHIT HE'S TOO FULL OF HIMSELF TO NOTICE.

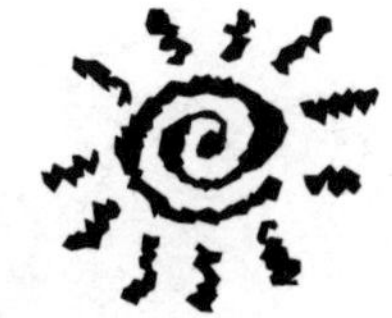

Why are men like lava lamps?

They are fun to look at but not all that bright.

HOW MANY MEN DOES IT TAKE TO CHANGE A LIGHT BULB?

NONE, THEY JUST SIT IN THE DARK AND COMPLAIN.

Why do married women weigh more than single women?

SINGLE WOMEN COME HOME,
CHECK WHAT'S IN THE FRIDGE
... AND GO TO BED.
MARRIED WOMEN COME HOME,
CHECK WHAT'S IN THE BED
... AND GO TO THE FRIDGE.

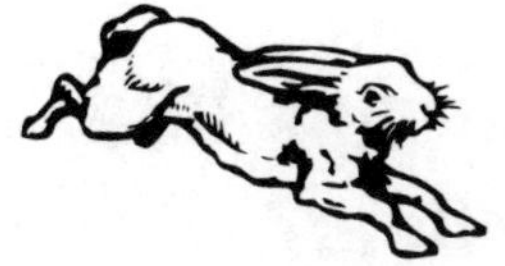

A man comes home from work with a packet of Olympic celebration condoms: one gold, one silver and one bronze.

'I think I'll use the gold one first,' he says to his girlfriend, 'because I'm the best.'

'Oh please,' she replies, 'can't you use the silver one? It would be nice if you came second for a change!'

WHY DO MEN NEVER BUY BUBBLE BATH?

THEY CAN JUST EAT BAKED BEANS FOR DINNER.

Why are most men like public toilets?

All the good ones are engaged and the only ones left are full of shit.

How can you tell a man is sexually aroused?

He's breathing.

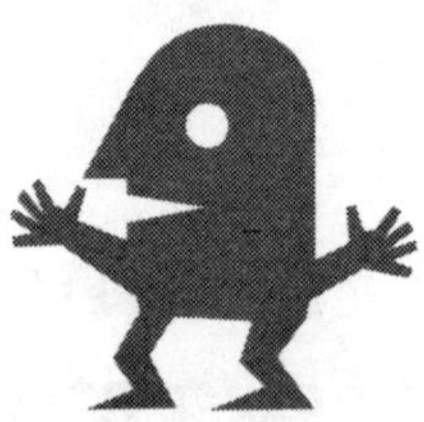

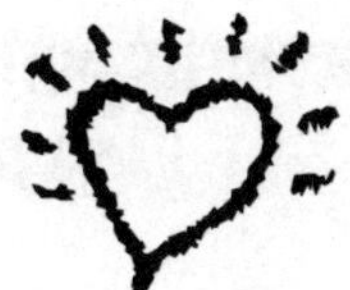

What's the quickest way to a man's heart?

Through his chest with a sharp knife.

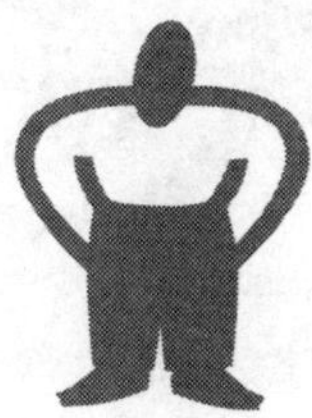

What's the difference between a new husband and a new dog?

After a year, the dog will still be excited to see you.

What do men have in common with beer bottles?

They are both empty from the neck up.

What is a man's favourite seven-course meal?

A six pack and a burger.

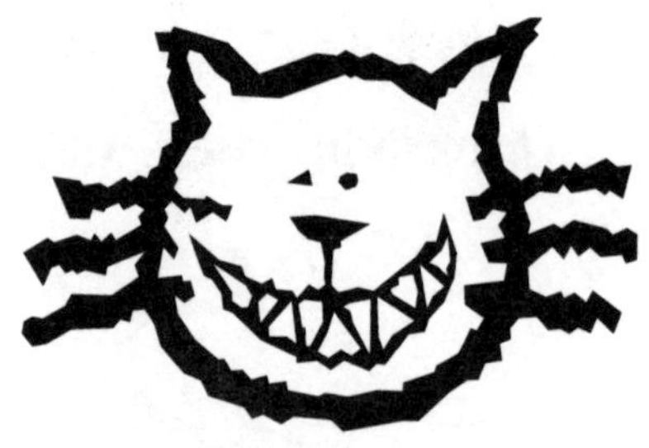

What do you call the useless piece of skin on the end of a penis?

A man.

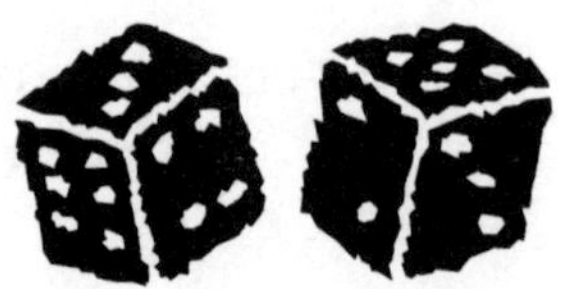

Why is e-mail like a man's dick?

It was created to transmit information vital to the survival of the species, but most people just use it for fun.

How do you know God is a man?

Because if God was a woman, semen would taste of chocolate.

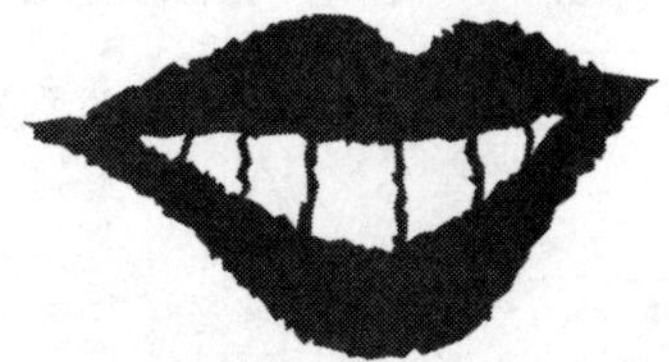

What can you do to get something hard and fast between your legs?

Buy a motorbike.

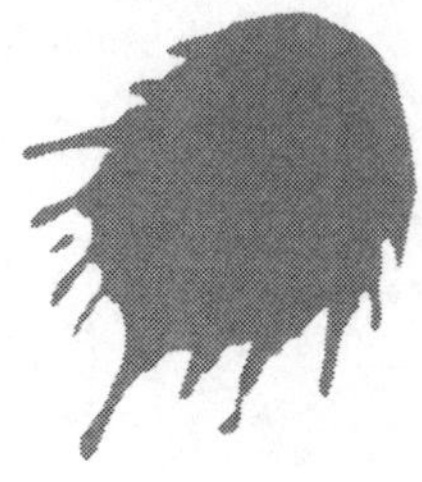

How many men does it take to wallpaper a bathroom?

Three – if you slice them very thinly.

What are a woman's three favourite animals?

A Jaguar in the garage,
a tiger in the bedroom, and
an ass to pay for it all.

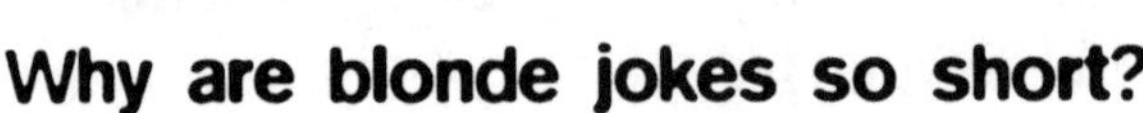

Why are blonde jokes so short?

So men can remember them.

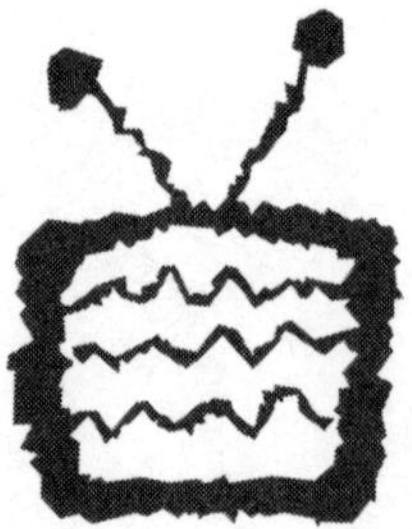

How do you get a man to do sit-ups to get rid of his beer gut?

Wedge the remote control between his toes.

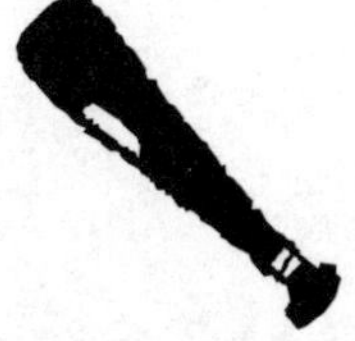

Why are men like cement?

They take a long time to get hard once they've been laid.

What do men have in common with a pair of tights?

They either cling, run or don't fit right in the crutch!

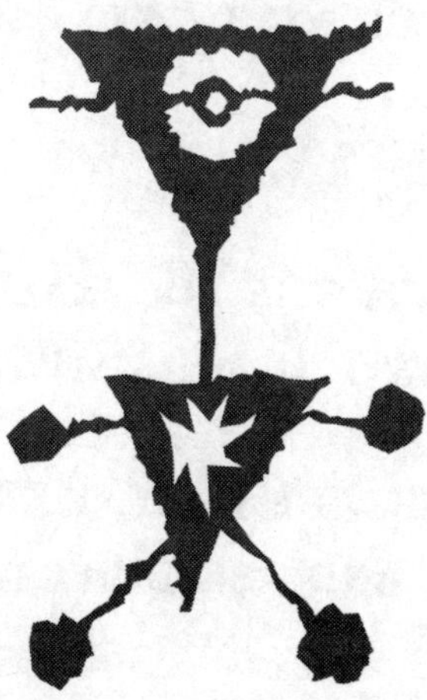

Seven Things you'll never hear from a Man

Her tits are just too big.

I think Mel Gibson is great looking.

I'd love to wear a condom.

While I'm up, can I get you a beer?

Sometimes I just want a hug.

Sod the football,
let's watch a slushy movie.

I think we are lost, we'd better
stop and ask directions.

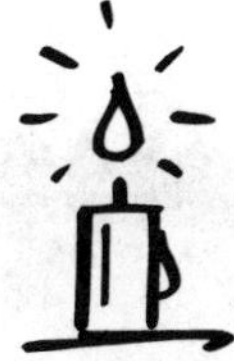

How many men does it take to screw in a light bulb?

One. He just holds it up there and waits for the world to revolve around him.

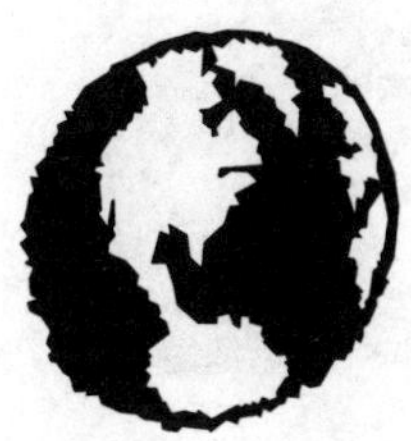

How can you tell when a man is well hung?

When you can't get your finger between his neck and the noose.

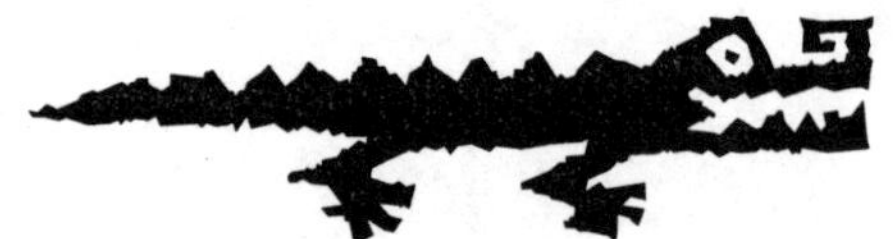

When would you care for a man's company?

When he owns it.

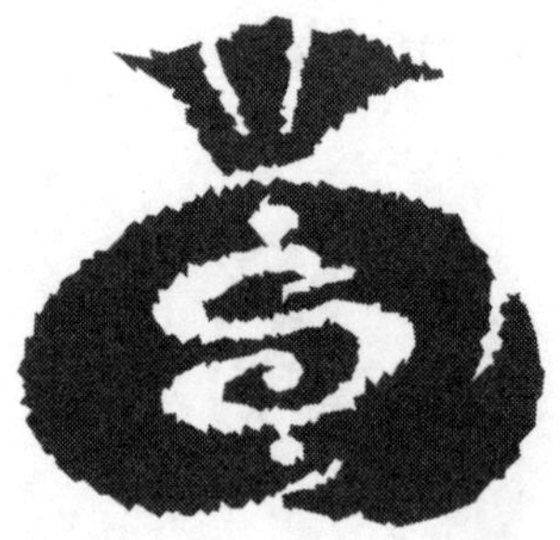

Why are men like savings accounts?

Without a lot of capital, they don't generate much interest.

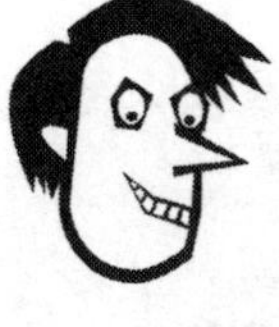

A man was intrigued to report some local gossip to his wife.

'They told me down at the pub that the milkman has slept with every woman in the street except one!'

'That'll be that snooty cow at number 35,' she replied.

What did the woman

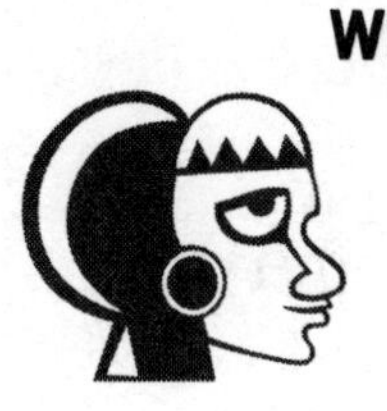

say to the guy who came up to her in the bar and said,

***'Hi, honey. What would you say to some ass?'*?**

'Goodbye ass.'

Why are men like holidays?

They never seem to be long enough.

An English professor wrote on the whiteboard:

'Woman without her man is nothing' and told the students to punctuate it.

The men wrote:
'Woman, without her man, is nothing.'

The women wrote:
'Woman! Without her, man is nothing.'

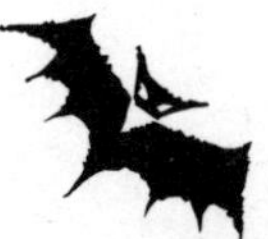

What's the difference between hard and dark?

It stays dark all night.

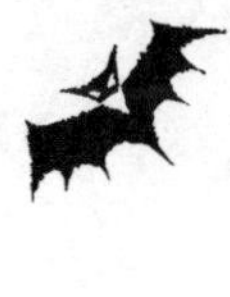

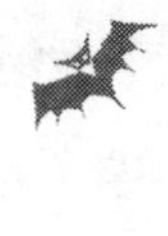

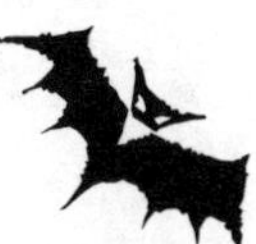

When a man says,
'Darling, we don't need material things
to prove our love,'
– he's forgotten your anniversary.

Why do men give names to their penises?

Because they don't like the idea of having a stranger make all their decisions.

What you do call a man doing the washing up?

A start.

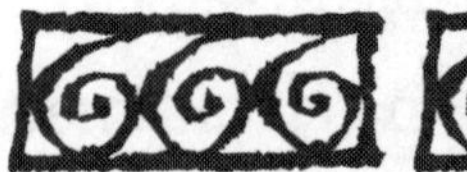
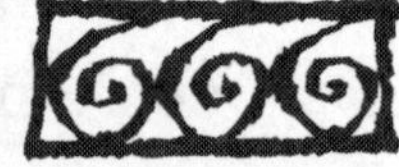

What is the male definition of commitment?

Not trying to pick up other women while he's out with you.

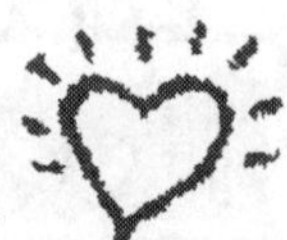

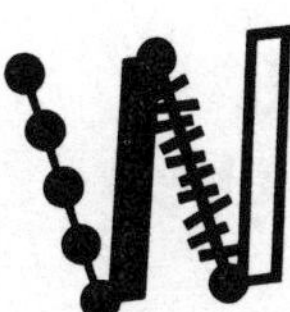

hy are the symptoms of stress like a perfect day?

They include eating too much chocolate,
impulse buying,
and driving far too fast.

W**hy do men like smart women?**

Opposites attract.

H**ow do you scare a man?**

Sneak up behind him and
start throwing rice.

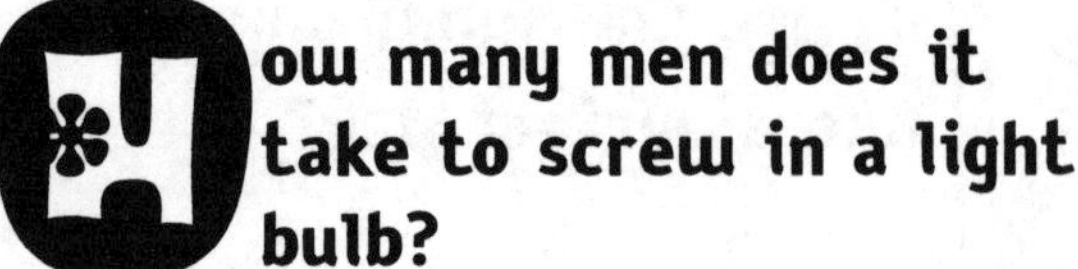

How many men does it take to screw in a light bulb?

Three. One to screw in the bulb and two to listen to him boasting about it.

Why are men like mini skirts?

If you're not careful, they'll creep up your legs.

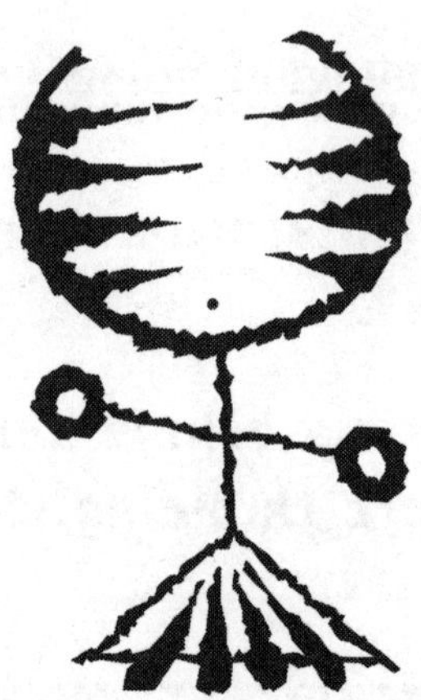

WHEN A MAN TELLS
HIS WIFE,
'I MISSED YOU,'
HE REALLY MEANS,
'I CAN'T FIND MY
SOCKS, THE KIDS ARE
HUNGRY AND WE ARE
OUT OF
TOILET PAPER.'

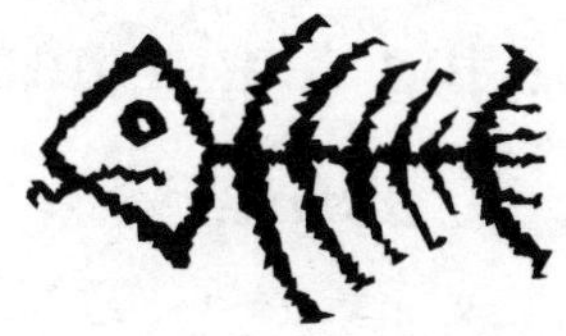

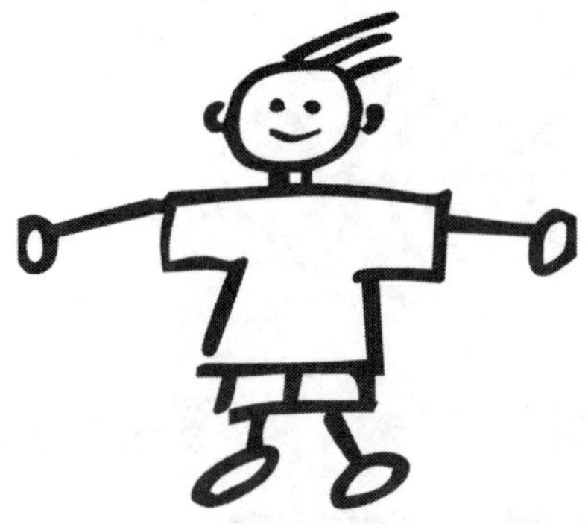

Why do little boys whine?

They are just practising for when they grow up.

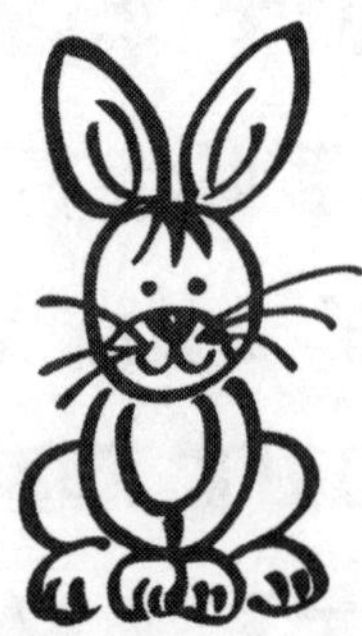

What do you call a man with 99% of his brain missing?

Castrated.

WHAT'S THE EASIEST WAY TO CONFUSE A MAN?

PUT A NAKED WOMAN AND A SIX-PACK IN FRONT OF HIM AND TELL HIM TO CHOOSE ONE.

How to impress a woman....

compliment her,
care for her,
respect her,
cuddle her,
kiss her,
caress her,
love her,
comfort her,
protect her,
trust her,
buy gifts for her,
wine and dine her,
listen to her,
stand by her,
support her.

How to impress a man...

show up naked,
bring beer.

Why do men get married?

Because they can't be bothered to hold their stomachs in any more.

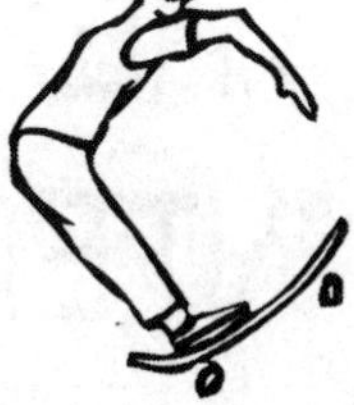

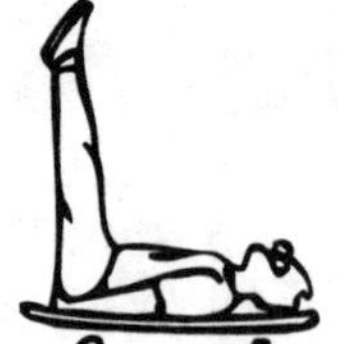

WHY ARE MEN LIKE ATM MACHINES?

ONCE THEY WITHDRAW, THEY LOSE INTEREST.

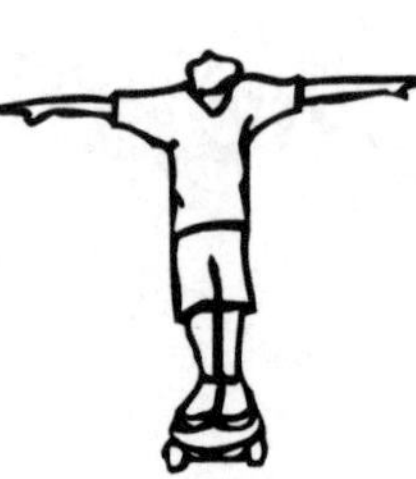

HOW DOES A MAN SHOW HE'S PLANNING FOR THE FUTURE?

HE BUYS TWO CASES OF BEER INSTEAD OF ONE.

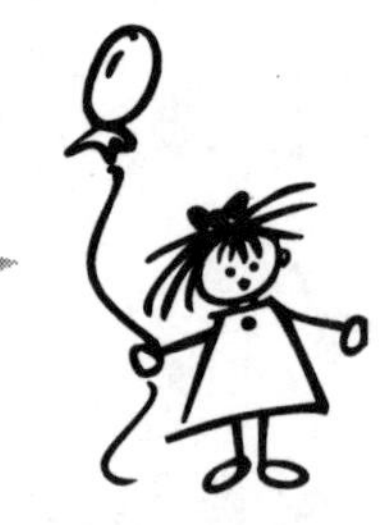

Women know all about their children: their friends, school times, dental appointments, favourite foods, secret fears and hopes and dreams—

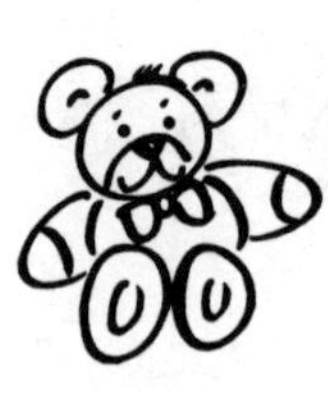

A man is vaguely aware of some short people living in the house.

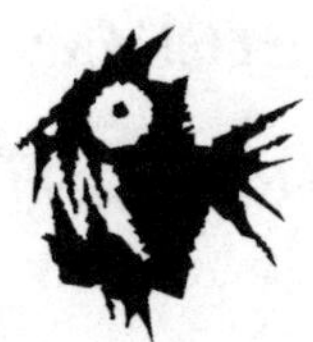
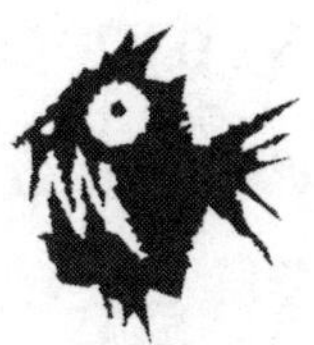
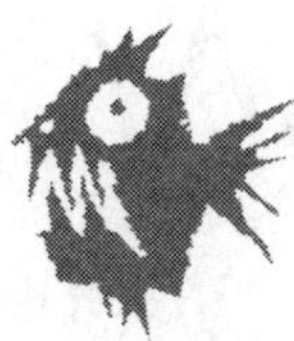

What's the difference between a man and a catfish?

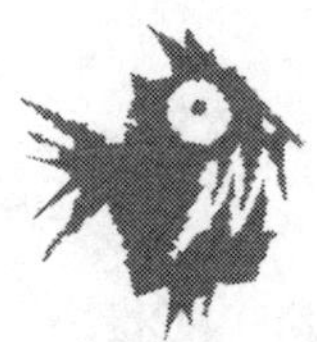
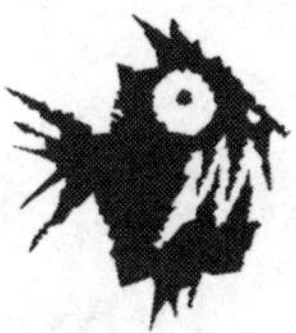
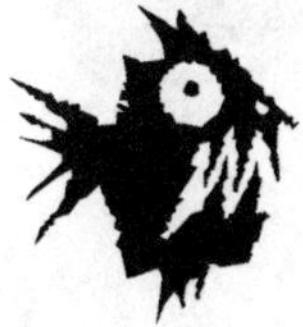

One's a bottom-feeding
scum-sucker...
and the other's a fish.

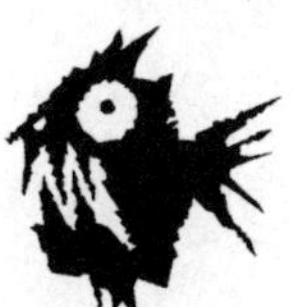
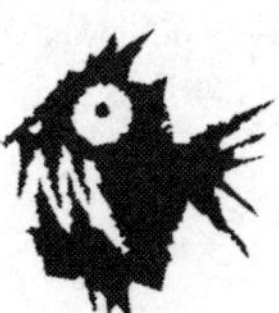
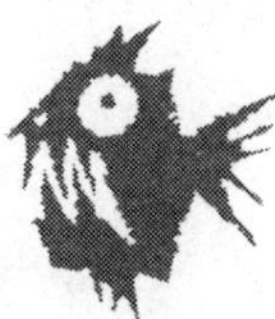

56

What's the difference between a man and yoghurt?

Yoghurt has culture.

How can you tell if you are having a super orgasm?

Your boyfriend wakes up.

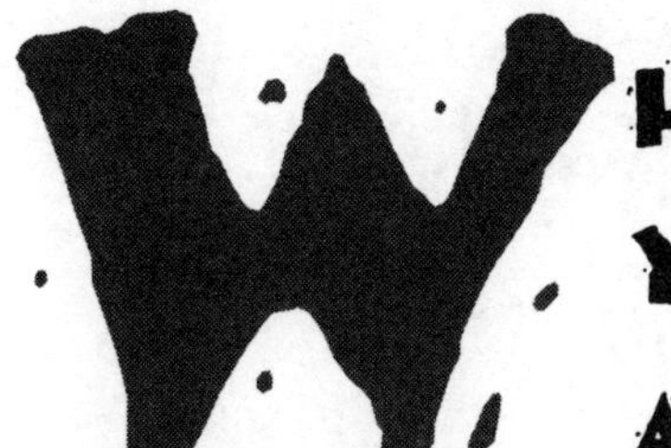

WHAT DO YOU CALL A MAN WHO SUPPORTS A WOMAN'S CAREER, IS AN EXCELLENT COOK, LOVES LOOKING AFTER THE KIDS AND EARNS A SIX-FIGURE INCOME?

DARLING.

What are a man's three favourite words to his partner?

'While you're up.'

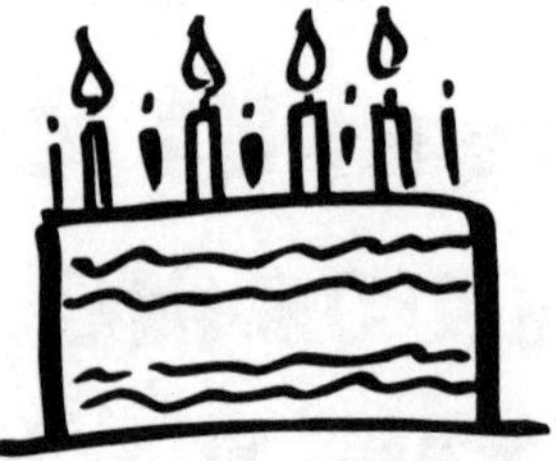

What do toilets and anniversaries have in common?

Men always miss them.

WHY ARE MEN LIKE COMPUTERS?

BECAUSE YOU ALWAYS HAVE TO TURN THEM ON TO GET THEIR ATTENTION.

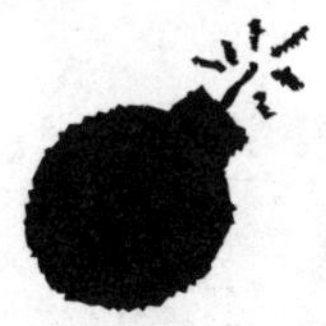

What's the difference between boring men and the M25 in the rush hour?

You can always turn off the motorway.

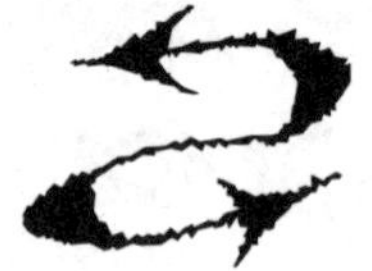

'My husband's an angel.'

'Lucky you. Mine's still alive.'

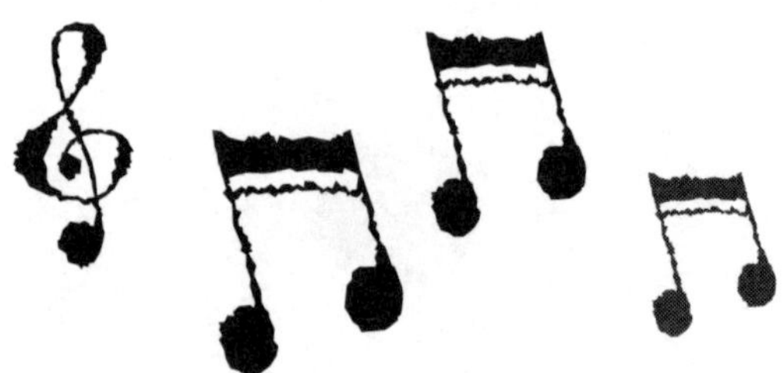

What do you call a man who can play the piano with no hands?

Clever Dick.

'I'm going to Belgium on holiday this year.'

'Antwerp?'

'No, he's staying at home.'

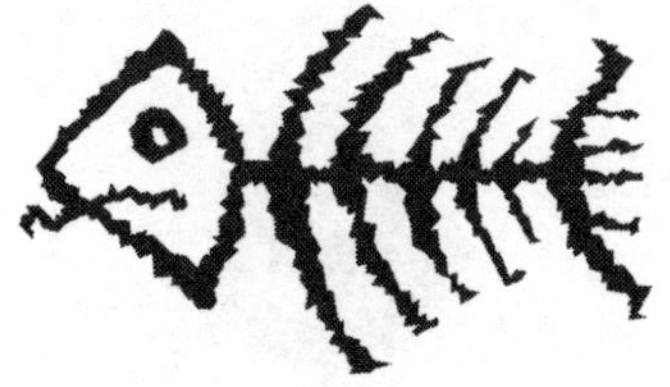

Why is food better than men?

You don't have to wait an hour for seconds.

What do you call men with an IQ of 180?

A village.

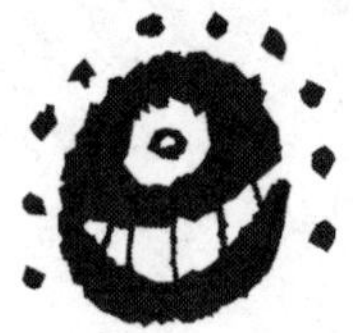

John was boasting that he was a knockout lover.

'I couldn't agree more,' said his girlfriend. 'Count to ten and it's all over!'

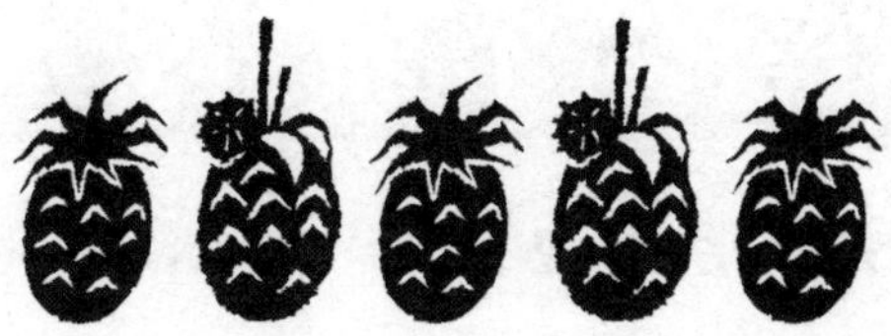

'Want a quickie?'

'As opposed to what?'

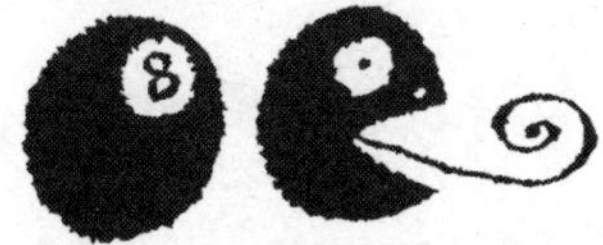

WHAT IS GROSS STUPIDITY?

144 MEN IN ONE ROOM.

Reasons why chocolate is better than sex

Good chocolate is easy to find.

'If you love me, you'll swallow' has real meaning with chocolate.

Chocolate satisfies even when it has gone soft.

If you bite the nuts too hard, the chocolate won't mind.

You can make chocolate last as long as you want it to.

You can have as many kinds of chocolate as you can handle.

With chocolate, size doesn't matter — it's always good.